MULTIPLE MYELOMA MANUAL

A Definitive step by step guide on the effective treatment for multiple myeloma

By

Dr. Harvey Donald

Copyright @ 2024

Table of Contents

PREFACE

This manual will specifically guide you on what you ought to know about multiple myeloma and its treatment. The book will guide you on signs and symptoms of multiple myeloma, causes and risk factors of multiple myeloma, complications of multiple myeloma, diagnosis and tests for multiple myeloma, stages of multiple myeloma, treatment for multiple myeloma, lifestyle tips and changes, multiple myeloma diet guide and so much more.

CHAPTER ONE

INTRODUCTION

Multiple myeloma is an uncommon form of cancer that affects the bone marrow as well as mutates or alters the blood's plasma cells. In other words, multiple myeloma occurs when healthy cells transform into abnormal cells that multiply and produce irregular antibodies referred to as *M proteins.* This change begins a cascade of medical problems and issues that can affect your bones, your kidneys and the capability of your body to produce healthy white and *red blood cells (erythrocytes) and platelets.*

Multiple myeloma is uncommon, thus affecting around 7 individuals out of 100,000 individuals per year. Healthcare professionals estimate around 100,000 individuals in the United

States of America have multiple myeloma.

Multiple myeloma which affects more men than women affects twice as many individuals who are black as it does individuals who are of other races. Majority of individuals with multiple myeloma are diagnosed between 40 and 70 years with the median age of diagnosis between 65 and 74 years.

*The plasma cells which are sometimes referred to as **B-cells** are a form and type of white blood cell as well as part of your immune system that are responsible for recognizing foreign infections as well as making antibodies to fight the foreign infections. These antibodies are referred to as **immunoglobins.***

*Plasma cells reside in your bone marrow; **the soft tissue that fills hollow bones** and in addition to plasma cells,* *bone marrow is also responsible for manufacturing other type of healthy blood cells.*

Multiple myeloma results into a buildup of cancer cells in your bone marrow with the cancer cells ultimately overtaking healthy blood cells which in turn unable your body to produce disease-fighting antibodies. Rather, it produces harmful proteins that impair your kidneys and give rise to other signs and symptoms.

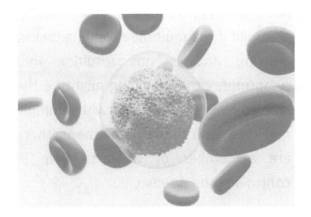

Some individuals have multiple myeloma without symptoms although

blood tests exhibit signs of conditions that may become multiple myeloma. In this case scenario, healthcare professionals may suggest watchful waiting or monitoring your general health instead of commencing treatment. Multiple myeloma cannot literally be cured by healthcare professionals, although related conditions and symptoms can be treated which in turn slow its progress.

Treatment for multiple myeloma is not always required immediately, although if the multiple myeloma is slow growing and is not resulting into symptoms, close watching might be the first step. For individuals with multiple myeloma who require treatment, there are a number of ways to help in controlling the disease.

CHAPTER TWO

SIGNS AND SYMPTOMS OF MULTIPLE MYELOMA

Some individuals don't have symptoms of multiple myeloma although tests exhibit they have conditions that may become multiple myeloma.

For instance, a **bone marrow aspiration or bone marrow biopsy** *may exhibit irregular or abnormal plasma cells and genetic mutations, which could entail you have* **smoldering multiple myeloma** *(an early onset precancerous type of multiple myeloma). Moreover, blood and urine tests may show proteins produced by abnormal plasma cells and this is a condition referred to as* **monoclonal gammopathy of undetermined significance.**

The symptoms of multiple myeloma develop in the course of time and may look like other medical conditions or diseases.

Some conditions connected to multiple myeloma and their causes include:

(a) **Bone Fracture/Bone Pain-** Bone pain and/or fracture can occur if abnormal or irregular plasma cells damage bone tissue, resulting into a soft spot in your bone. These are referred to as *osteolytic lesions.*

(b) **Anemia-** You don't have sufficient red blood cells (erythrocytes) since multiplying abnormal plasma cells don't allow room for your red blood cells.

(c) **Thrombocytopenia-** You don't have sufficient platelets (*the cells that help your blood clot)* due to the fact that abnormal plasma cells crowd out those platelets and keep your bone marrow from producing sufficient platelets.

(d) **Kidney issues/failure:** Your kidneys filter waste and toxins, although abnormal plasma cells make ***M proteins*** that block the filtering process which in turn impair your kidneys. *Note that myeloma cells produce harmful proteins that can result into kidney damage as well as kidney failure.*

(e) **Hypercalcemia-** Hypercalcemia occurs when impaired or debilitated bones release excess calcium into your bloodstream.

(f) **Amyloidosis-** Amyloidosis occurs when abnormal proteins (amyloid proteins) accumulate in your organs.

(g) Hyperviscosity syndrome- *M proteins (proteins produced by abnormal plasma cells)* thicken your blood thus making your heart to work harder to pump blood all through your body.

(h) Bacterial infection, specifically pneumonia- Like red blood cells, abnormal or irregular plasma cells are multiplying and clogging healthy white blood cells (erythrocytes) that resist or fight infection.

(i) Cryoglobulinemia- Proteins in your blood can cluster together when it is cold as a result of multiple myeloma.

Multiple myeloma and its symptoms

Early in multiple myeloma, there might be no symptoms although multiple myeloma causes numerous symptoms with *bone pain* being usually the first symptom individuals observe. Some of the other symptoms of multiple myeloma may include:

(a) Bone pain, particularly in the chest, spine, or hips.

(b) Having fatigue and feeling weak- Healthy cells allow your body to fight invading germs easily and as myeloma cells replaces bone marrows; your bone has to work much harder with fewer disease-fighting cells which in turn make you tire more easily. *Having fatigue and a feeling of weakness is a sign of anemia (low red blood count).*

(c) Weakness in your arms and legs as well as a sensation of numbness in your arms and legs. Multiple myeloma can as well affect the bones in your spine thus resulting into collapse and press on your spinal cord.

(d) Nausea and vomiting which may also be a sign of hypercalcemia (high blood calcium levels).

(e) Unexplained loss of weight

(f) Constipation

(g) Needing to urinate more often than normal

(h) Infections- As a result of fewer antibodies in your blood, fighting infections becomes more difficult.

(i) Dizziness

(j) Lack of appetite as well as feeling thirstier than normal. These are also signs of high blood calcium levels (hypercalcemia).

(k) Unexplained fever which may be a symptom of a *bacterial infection.*

(l) Bleeding more easily or bruising which may be a sign of abnormal plasma cells which in turn prevent your body from producing adequate platelets.

(m)   Unexplained confusion or *mental fogginess.*

Myeloma cells crowd out healthy blood cells thus resulting into low red blood counts (anemia) as well as low white blood counts (leucopenia).

CHAPTER THREE

CAUSES AND RISK FACTORS OF MULTIPLE MYELOMA

Healthcare professionals and physicians are still unsure of the precise cause of multiple myeloma, although it is known that multiple myeloma involves changes in the genes that are control plasma cell growth and division.

The most prevalent genetic mutations are **tumor suppressor genes** *such as p53 genes,* **Oncogenes** *such as RAS and MYC, and Deletion of chromosome number 17.*

Dendritic cells in bone marrow can also result into multiple myeloma as they release a hormone referred to as interleukin-6 (IL-6) to induce growth in plasma cells. Nevertheless, excess production of interleukin-6 can promote abnormal cell growth and an elevated risk for plasma cell tumors.

Potential causes of multiple myeloma may include:

(a) **Environmental Factors-** Some studies have been able to demonstrate potential links between multiple myeloma and exposure to radiation or chemicals in pesticides.

(b) **Having an inflammatory disease or medical condition-** Inflammatory diseases may include *Type 2 diabetes, rheumatoid arthritis and heart disease.*

(c) **Having obesity-** Having high levels of body fat can also result into multiple myeloma

(d) **Genetic mutations-** Links between mutating or changing oncogenes and multiple myeloma are currently being investigated by healthcare professionals and researchers. It is also deduced that most individuals who have multiple myeloma don't have all pieces of *chromosome number 17.*

Risk Factors

Multiple myeloma begins with a condition referred to as ***monoclonal gammopathy of undetermined significance,*** also known as **MGUS.** Furthermore, in MGUS, the level of ***M proteins*** in the blood is low, although the M proteins don't cause damage in the body.

Various factors elevate the risk of developing multiple myeloma and they include:

(a) **Race-** African Americana are more likely to develop multiple myeloma as Caucasians.

(b) **Obesity/overweight-** Research demonstrates that obesity during early and late stage of adulthood elevates the risk of developing multiple myeloma.

(c) **Age-** The risk of developing multiple myeloma increases with age. Most individuals who receive a diagnosis for multiple myeloma are often in their mid-60s **(65 to 74 years)**. Less than 1% of individuals diagnosed with multiple myeloma are younger than 55 and this is according to the *American Cancer Society.*

(d) **Sex-** Men are at a higher chance of developing this type of cancer than women.

(e) **Family History-** You are more likely to be diagnosed with myeloma if you have a sibling or parent with the condition. Nevertheless, family history only accounts for a small fraction of myeloma cases.

(f) **Monoclonal gammopathy of undetermined significance (MGUS) –** In nearly all cases, multiple myeloma starts as a benign condition referred to as *monoclonal gammopathy of undetermined significance (MGUS),* along with low levels of monoclonal proteins otherwise referred to as M proteins.

(g) Exposure to radiation

(h) Contact with chemicals used in rubber manufacturing, woodworking, or firefighting/or in herbicides.

There is literally no way to prevent myeloma and if you get or develop multiple myeloma, you did not do anything to cause it.

CHAPTER FOUR

COMPLICATIONS OF MULTIPLE MYELOMA AND ITS TREATMENT

As multiple myeloma progresses or develops further, it can somewhat result into complications such as:

(a) **Bone Problems/Pain-** Bone pain, debilitated or thinning bones as well as broken bones are all prevalent and common complications of multiple myeloma.

(b) **Anemia-** Normal blood cells will be crowded or pushed out of your bone marrow and replaced by cancer cells, which can result into anemia and other blood issues or blood problems.

(c) **Regular or frequent infections-** As myeloma cells crowd out healthy plasma cells, your body will then lack the capability to fight against infections.

(d) Decreased Kidney function- M proteins which are harmful antibodies produced by the myeloma cancer cells can damage your kidneys, cause problems with kidney function, and ultimately result into kidney failure. Furthermore, damaged and nibbling bones can elevate your blood's calcium levels and these high levels of calcium can interfere with your kidneys' capability to filter waste.

Treatment of multiple myeloma might include treating its complications.

(a) Infections- Infections such as the *flu and pneumonia* can be prevented by vaccines.

(b) Bone Pain- Bone pain can be controlled by pain medications, surgery as well as radiation therapy.

(c) **Kidney damages/reduced kidney function-** Individuals with severe kidney damage may require dialysis.

(d) **Anemia-** Medications can increase the number of red blood cells **(erythrocytes)** in the blood as this can help relieve ongoing anemia.

(e) **Bone loss-** Bone-building medications might help in preventing loss of bone.

CHAPTER FIVE

DIAGNOSIS AND TESTS FOR MULTIPLE MYELOMA

If cancer is suspected, your physician may order various imaging tests such as MRI scan, CT scan, positron emission, PET scan, or a bone X-ray to confirm its presence as well as show bone problems connected with multiple myeloma. Multiple myeloma is often diagnosed when there is a confirmation of a plasma cell tumor or a minimum of 10% of plasma cells in the bone marrow.

Furthermore, it is also required by physicians to find at least one of the following symptoms such as:

(a) Elevated levels of light chains
(b) 60% or more plasma cells in the bone marrow as well as tumor with holes in the bones

(c) Low red blood cell counts (anemia) as well as poor kidney function.

Blood tests and urine tests are one of the first tools for diagnosing multiple myeloma and these can include:

(a) Blood chemistry tests
(b) Serum free light chains
(c) Beta-2 microglobuin
(d) Electrophoresis
(e) Several types of urine tests
(f) Quantitative immunoglobulins and complete blood counts.

BLOOD TESTS- The M proteins made by myeloma cells can appear or show up in a blood sample. Blood cells might also find another protein myeloma cells make, which is referred to as **beta-2 microglobulin.** Other blood tests may give a clue about your diagnosis and some of these tests might include tests that look at kidney function, blood cell counts as well as levels of calcium and uric acid.

URINE TESTS- M proteins can appear in urine samples and in urine samples, the proteins are referred to as *Bence Jones proteins.*

A biopsy which involves taking a tissue sample from the tumor, lymph node, or bone marrow can also be used in diagnosing multiple myeloma.

Some of the common biopsies used in diagnosing this type of cancer may include:

(a) Fine needle aspiration
(b) Core needle biopsy
(c) Bone marrow biopsy/Bone marrow aspiration.

Bone Marrow Biopsy/Bone Marrow Tests- Bone marrow biopsy and bone marrow aspiration are used in collecting bone marrow samples for diagnosis. Bone marrow contains a solid and a liquid part and again, in a bone marrow biopsy, a needle is used in collecting a little amount of the solid tissue. In a bone marrow aspiration, a needle is used in drawing a sample of the fluid with samples generally taken from the hip bone.

The samples will then go to a laboratory in order to test or diagnose for multiple myeloma cells. Other special tests offer your health care team additional information about your myeloma cells. For instance, the fluorescence in situ hybridization test checks for alterations in the cells' genetic material, referred to as DNA.

STAGES/STAGING

As soon as your physician has confirmed a test or diagnosis of multiple myeloma, the next step is to see how far it has spread in the body. Multiple myeloma is grouped into three (3) various stages and each stage can ascertain an individual's survival rate and treatment choices.

An individual in Stage 1will have:

(a) Serum beta-2 microglobulin less than 3.5 mg/L
(b) Albumin level equal to or higher than 3.5g/Dl
(c) Bone marrow tests or diagnosis do not group as high risk.
(d) Normal LDH (Lactate dehydrogenase) levels

Physicians may group you as **Stage 2** if you do not fall into the criteria for **stage 1 or stage 3.**

An individual in Stage 3 will have:

(a) Serum beta-2 microglobulin equal to or higher than 5.5mg/L
(b) Bone marrow biopsies or Bone marrow tests group a patient as high risk.
(c) High LDH (Lactate dehydrogenase) levels.

The results of your tests and diagnosis help the health care professionals to decide your stage of myeloma and in multiple myeloma, the stages vary from 1 to 3. The stage describes your health care professionals how quickly your myeloma is growing. A Stage 1 multiple myeloma is growing gradually and as the stages gets higher, the myeloma becomes more combative. A Stage 3 multiple myeloma is getting aggravated instantly. Multiple myeloma can also be given a risk level and this is another way to say how combative this type of cancer is. Your healthcare team makes use of the multiple myeloma stage and risk level to determine your diagnosis and map out your treatment.

CHAPTER SIX

TREATMENT FOR MULTIPLE MYELOMA

Unlike healthy, normal cells, cancer cells do not fully develop and function effectively, or undergo apoptosis (entailing they die away when they are no longer required). Rather, they live and accumulate and in the case of multiple myeloma, cancer cells quickly multiply and ultimately submerging bone marrow.

The production of cancer cells surpasses the production of healthy blood cells, and the cancer cells oust the healthy ones. This results into *fatigue, anemia,* and regular infections.

Rather than producing beneficial antibodies just like normal plasma cells, myeloma cancer cells produce abnormal and toxic antibodies. Your body can't make use of these antibodies, referred to as *monoclonal proteins, or M proteins.* These proteins accumulate in your body and harm your kidneys overtime.

Multiple myeloma is generally not curable and patients usually require numerous treatment options over the course of their illness, especially as some treatments may stop working and new ones will require to be engaged. There are numerous drug therapies available to control symptoms, kill multiple myeloma cells, and reduce the spread of the cancer.

Multiple myeloma treatment is not regularly required immediately and if there are no symptoms, you might have tests to watch the myeloma to see if it gets aggravated. When multiple myeloma results into symptoms, treatment usually begins with medications. Treatment usually helps in easing pain, controlling complications as well as reducing the growth of the myeloma cells.

Multiple myeloma does not result into symptoms occasionally and this is usually referred to as *smoldering multiple myeloma.*

If the myeloma is at an early stage and is growing gradually, you might have frequent checkups to keep a check on the cancer. A health care professional or a physician might test your blood and urine to check for signs that the myeloma is getting aggravated.

Furthermore, you and your health care professionals might choose to begin treatment if you develop symptoms of multiple myeloma.

Immunotherapy- Immunotherapy is a treatment with medications that helps the body's immune system to destroy cancer cells. The immune system resists or fights off diseases by invading germs and other cells that should not be in the body. Cancer cells thrive by hiding from the immune system with immunotherapy helping immune system cells find and destroy the cancer cells.

(a) **Targeted Therapy-** Targeted therapy makes use of medications that invade specific chemicals in the cancer cells and by blocking these chemicals, targeted treatments can kill the cancer cells.

(b) **Corticosteroids-** Corticosteroid medications helps in controlling irritation and swelling referred to as *inflammation* in the body. Furthermore, corticosteroids also help in fighting off myeloma cells.

Furthermore, steroids also help in reducing side effects from chemotherapy such as *nausea and vomiting*. **Prednisone and dexamethasone** are two (2) prescribed steroids that at high doses can decrease the number of myeloma cells.

(c) **Chemotherapy-** Chemotherapy makes use of strong medications to fights off cancer cells with the medications destroying fast-growing cells such as *myeloma cells.*

(d) **CAR-T cell therapy (Chimeric antigen receptor T cell therapy) –** The CAR-T cell therapy which trains your immune system cells to fight against multiple myeloma begins with removing some white blood cells, such as T cells from your blood with the blood cells then sent to a laboratory. The cells are then treated in the lab so that they make special receptors. The receptors help the cells in identifying a marker on the surface of the myeloma cells and then the cells are put back into the body as they can now find and kill the multiple myeloma cells.

(e) **Radiation Therapy-** Radiation therapy makes use of strong or powerful energy beams to destroy cancer cells. The energy usually emerges from X-rays, protons or other sources. Radiation which can instantly shrink a growth of myeloma cells might be used if myeloma cells form a mass referred to as *plasmacytoma.* Radiation may help in controlling or regulating a plasmacytoma that is causing pain or impairing a bone.

(f) **Monoclonal antibodies-** Enhance your immune system by bringing in antibodies that target specific proteins on myeloma cells.

(g) **Proteasome inhibitors-** Kills cancer cells by stopping them from getting rid of old proteins.

(h) **Immunomodulatory drugs-** Stimulates or activates immune cells to help in detecting and disposing myeloma cells.

(i) **HDAC (Histone deacetylase inhibitors) –** Drugs that represses the cell cycle and prevent cancer cells from growing as well as dividing.

(j) **Bone marrow transplant-** A Bone marrow transplant, also referred to as a *stem cell transplant,* replaces weak bone marrow with strong bone marrow.

Prior to a bone marrow transplant, blood-forming stem

cells are collected from your blood and then high doses of chemotherapy are administered to kill your diseased or weak bone marrow. The stem cells are then put into your body as they travel to the bones and start rebuilding bone marrow. This form of transplant using your own cells is referred to as an **autologous bone marrow transplant.**

The stem cells occasionally come from a healthy donor. This form of transplant is referred to as an **allergic bone marrow transplant.**

Your treatment plan will usually depend on whether you are likely to have a bone marrow transplant and when deciding if bone marrow transplant is the best option for you, your healthcare professionals considers numerous factors and these factors may include whether your multiple myeloma is likely to get aggravated, your age as well as your general health.

If your healthcare professionals thinks or decides that bone marrow transplant is an excellent option for you, treatment usually starts with a mix of medications. The mix might include corticosteroids, immunotherapy, chemotherapy as well as targeted therapy. After a few months of treatment, blood stem cells are usually collected from your blood and then bone marrow transplant might occur soon after collecting the cells. Although you might hold on or wait after a relapse particularly if there is one. Sometimes, physicians suggest two bone marrow transplants for individuals with multiple myeloma.

After the bone marrow transplant, you will likely have immunotherapy or targeted therapy as these can help in keeping the myeloma from emerging again or coming back.

When bone marrow transplant is not an option or if you decide not to have a bone marrow transplant, treatment might include a mix of medications and the mix might include corticosteroids, immunotherapy, chemotherapy, as well as targeted therapy.

Furthermore, treatment might involve having another course of the same treatment particularly when myeloma comes back or does not respond to treatment.

CHAPTER SEVEN

MULTIPLE MYELOMA DIET GUIDE

If you are diagnosed with multiple myeloma, the side effects of chemotherapy may cause you to lose your appetite, skip meals on a regular schedule thus causing your body to lack vital nutrients.

Maintaining excellent nutrition is vital, particularly while you are undergoing treatment. Multiple myeloma can leave you with decreased immunity, damaged kidneys, as well as anemia. Nevertheless, some simple diet tips can help you in feeling better as well as offering you the strength to fight back.

Although there is no specific diet you must follow when you have multiple myeloma, some *nutritional strategies* may help decrease common symptoms, support your health, as well as keep you strong and healthy while undergoing treatment. Consuming small amount of meals throughout the day that are rich in fruits, proteins, and vegetables can help nourish your body and enhance your general health and well-being.

BENEFITS OF EATING A HEALTHY DIET FOR MULTIPLE MYELOMA

Consuming a healthy diet may help in enhancing or improving symptoms of multiple myeloma. Eating well may also help in relieving some psychological symptoms such as anxiety and depression that many individuals with multiple myeloma can experience.

Eating well ensures you get the vital nutrients your body requires to enhance your immunity, boost your strength as well as positively impact your general health and well-being.

1. **Enhance/Boost immune system-** Cancer and chemotherapy treatments can debilitate your immune system, thus making you more prone to falling sick. Fruits and vegetables comprise of vitamins and minerals such as *vitamins C and E* that can help enhance immune function and decrease the risk of falling sick.

Practicing food safety can also help in decreasing your risk of infection. Wash your hands prior to handling food, stay away from individuals that are sick, and ensure all meats are cooked properly before eating. Do well to stay clear of *raw eggs, sushi, and other raw foods (apart from fruits and veggies),* which may carry bacteria and viruses that can make you fall sick.

When your immunity is decreased, fruits and veggies that have not been peeled can constitute a risk to your health. Cooking your food to the minimum recommended internal temperatures destroys any bacteria that may be present and can help prevent you from having a food-borne illness.

2. **Enhance kidney health-** Multiple myeloma can lead to kidney damage in some individuals and as the cancer crowds out healthy blood cells, it can result into a breakdown of bone. This is important due to the fact that your bones release calcium into your blood.

When you have kidney damage, waste and fluid can accumulate in the body, thus resulting into stress on essential organs.

A kidney-friendly diet means you avoid certain foods and minerals to protect your kidneys as this will help in preventing waste and fluid from accumulating in the body, causing further damage.

To help in protecting your kidneys, it is vital you track your intake of fat, salt, alcohol, potassium, protein, carbohydrate as well as sodium as these can overwork your kidneys.

The amount of water and other fluids you drink may have to be limited if your kidneys are severely damages and also you may need to consume less calcium if your blood calcium levels are high since portions of your bone are destroyed from the cancer. Consult your physician before making any dietary changes as a result of kidney disease.

3. **Fiber for Balance and regularity-** Chemotherapy and some chemotherapy drugs can sometimes result into constipation. Increasing your soluble (dissolvable) fiber intake can help with the frequency and ease of bowel movements which in turn prevent constipation.

   Some of the foods that are high and rich in fiber may include:

   (a) Berries

   (b) Beans, nuts, and lentils.

(c) Broccoli, artichokes, and carrots

(d) Dried fruits *such as figs, prunes, apricots and raisins*

(e) Whole grains *such as brown rice and oatmeal.*

(f) Pears, oranges, and apples

Increasing your intake of water may also help in keeping things moving in your digestive system. Prune juice can also play a vital role if you are constipated.

4. **Decrease inflammation-** *Curcumin,* the active ingredient in the spice turmeric, has powerful anti-inflammatory and anti-cancer effects with a 2021 study demonstrating that *curcumin*

may help in slowing the growth of cancerous cells.

Numerous patients with multiple myeloma experience a relapse *(return of multiple myeloma)* as a result of acquired multidrug resistance.

Studies have demonstrated that curcumin supplementation may decrease the risk of becoming resistant to some chemotherapy drugs and may even reverse acquired multidrug resistance.

Numerous individuals with multiple myeloma find bland foods easier to consume. Try adding turmeric to your meals if you can and again some foods such as *cheeses, mustard, and ghee* contain turmeric.

5. **Boost Red Blood cell count-** Anemia or a low red blood cell count is a prevalent complication in individuals with multiple myeloma. When cancerous plasma cells in your blood proliferate, there is not adequate room for your red blood cells. Basically, the cancer cells crowd out and kill the healthy ones.

A low red blood cell count can result into several problems such as *fatigue, weakness and cold sensation.*

Low levels of iron in your blood can also result into anemia and if you have developed anemia as a result of multiple myeloma, your physician may suggest you consume more foods containing iron. A boost in iron levels can help you less fatigued as well as help your body in making more healthy red blood cells (erythrocytes).

Some excellent sources of iron may include *kale, sweet potatoes, bell peppers, brussel sprouts, broccoli, raisins, lean red meat, and tropical fruits (papaya, mango, guava, and papaya).*

How Multiple Myeloma Diet Works

Living with multiple myeloma can make it hard to eat as a result of the symptoms of blood cancer and side effects of treatment.

Some of the steps to help ensure you get the right nutrition that will help you in regaining your strength and feeling better may include:

(a) Eating foods that are easy on your stomach.

(b) Consuming a range of fruits and vegetables.

(c) Consuming small and more frequent meals all through the day.

(d) Consuming more of protein-rich foods and limiting processed foods and sugars.

(e) Drinking plenty of fluids specifically *water*.

(f) Practicing food safety such as *ensuring your meats are thoroughly cooked and sanitizing your hands before handling foods.*

Consuming healthy foods rich in nutrients can be a lifelong journey, even after you have completed treatment for multiple myeloma and again, consuming a balanced diet offers a host of health benefits that will help your general health and well-being.

Furthermore, always consult your healthcare professional before starting a new diet, especially when undergoing treatment. Your healthcare team may suggest you consult a dietitian, who can help you in coming up with a diet strategy to ensure your body acquires all the nutrients it requires while going through cancer treatment.

Foods to eat on the Multiple Myeloma diet

When following a multiple myeloma diet, you will focus on consuming nutrient-dense foods while decreasing your intake of processed foods, sugars, and refined carbohydrates.

Some of the recommended foods may include:

(a) Asparagus
(b) Apples

(c) Broccoli

(d) Lean meats

(e) Leafy green vegetables

(f) Lentils

(g) Eggs

(h) Pears

(i) Fish

(j) Yogurts

(k) Crackers

(l) Potatoes

(m)   Nuts

(n) Whole grains such as *brown rice, oatmeal.*

*Consuming plenty of **fruits and vegetables,** which are rich in antioxidants and important vitamins and minerals, can enhance your immune system, keep your bowel movements regular, and improve your energy levels.*

Lean proteins such as lentils, beans, white-fleshed fish, and chicken help your body in building your skin, muscle, and hair. Furthermore, lean proteins also help the body in building antibodies to keep your immune system healthy and strong.

Nuts are rich in fiber and healthy fats, which in turn helps in decreasing inflammation and keep your bowels moving.

Try consuming small amount of meals throughout the day to ensure you get sufficient calories and nutrition. Multiple myeloma and cancer treatments tend to decrease your appetite, and thus it is vital to eat when you can.

Foods to avoid on the Multiple Myeloma diet

(a) Alcohol
(b) Raw meat
(c) Runny eggs
(d) Sushi

(e) Soda and other sugar-sweetened drinks

(f) Unwashed veggies and fruits

(g) Foods rich in potassium such as *avocados, citrus fruits and bananas*

(h) Foods rich and high in sodium such as *processed foods, sauces, and packaged snacks*

(i) Desserts made and prepared with processed sugars such as *baked goods.*

Multiple Myeloma cooking tips and dietary restrictions

Multiple myeloma and cancer treatments can have an impact on your immune system, thus making you more prone to infection. Practicing good food safety is vital to keep your body healthy and some recommendations may include:

(a) Washing your hands before handling food

(b) Making use of separate knives and cutting boards for meats and fruits and vegetables.

(c) Cooking all your foods to their correct temperature and ensuring all meat is properly cooked.

Numerous individuals with multiple myeloma find it easier to consume and digest bland foods and thus eat what you can and add spices only when you feel your stomach can tolerate it.

Your dietary options can make a large impact on your physical and emotional health. Foods are vital in keeping your body healthy, and thus try eating as many nutrient-dense foods as you can when you have an appetite.

If you are not acquainted to following a specific diet, it can be somewhat difficult to consume whole, unprocessed foods at first. Change can be difficult, but instead of concentrating on what you can't eat, think about how your dietary changes will help you better cope with stress and feel stronger and healthier. It is vital to eat healthy, fresh foods more often than not.

Aim to eat as many whole, fresh foods as you can as you will want to decrease your intake of processed foods whenever possible. Try cutting down on eating uncooked or cured meats, fast food, packaged snacks, and other processed foods that are rich in sodium, sugar, as well as starches. Reduce your intake of alcohol and sugar-sweetened drinks.

CONCLUSION

Multiple myeloma is a form of cancer that is not curable, although it is treatable. An individual who receives a diagnosis has a chance of living at least another 5 years. About 4.8% of individuals receive a diagnosis in the early stages. Getting some physical exercise, adequate rest, finding a local support group to help with emotional and other help, stopping smoking, if appropriate are some of the lifestyle changes that help in managing multiple myeloma. Nevertheless, any individual with multiple myeloma should consult their physician before attempting an alternative or complementary therapy, as some remedies can interact with existing treatments which in turn aggravate symptoms.

THE END

Made in United States
Troutdale, OR
06/26/2024

20832551R00037